KETO COOKIES

Discover 30 Easy to Follow Ketogenic Cookbook Cookies recipes for Your Low-Carb Diet with Gluten-Free and wheat to Maximize your weight loss

STEPHANIE BAKER

Copyright © Stephanie Baker

All rights reserved. No part of this book may be reproduced, scanned or distributed in any printed or electronic form without permission. Please do not participate in or encourage piracy of copyrighted materials in violation of the author's rights. Purchase only authorized editions.

1

LOW CARB SESAME TALER (FAKE OATMEAL COOKIES)

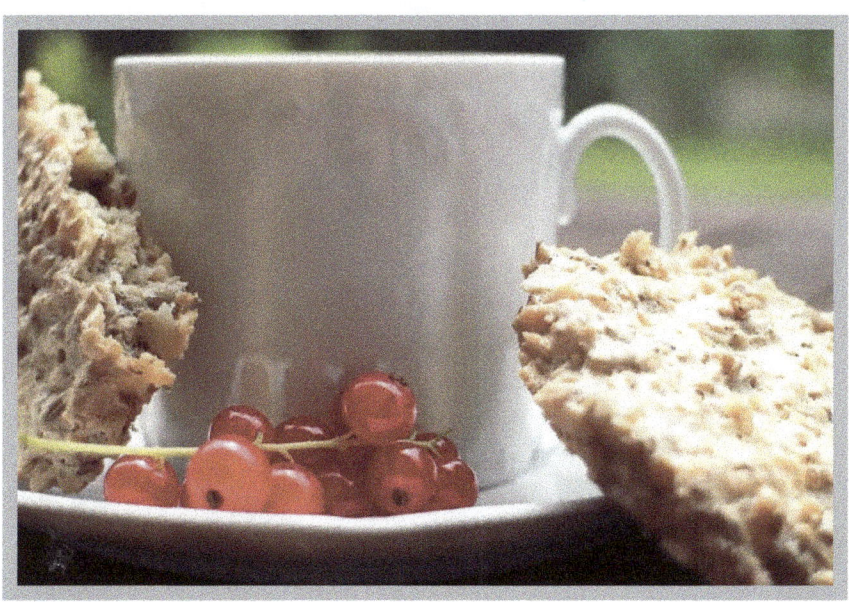

INGREDIENTS

PREPARATION

Preheat the oven to 150 ° C.

Whisk the egg whites vigorously by pouring the xylitol.

If necessary, mash the almonds and mix them with the sesame seeds, sunflower seeds and chopped hazelnuts.

Add the nut mixture to the egg white.

We form the mixture into nine thalers with the help of a spoon and place on a baking sheet lined with parchment paper.

Cook for 15 minutes until golden brown.

Preparation time: about 25 minutes.

SERVINGS: about 9 thalers.

2
LOW-CARB FLORENTINES

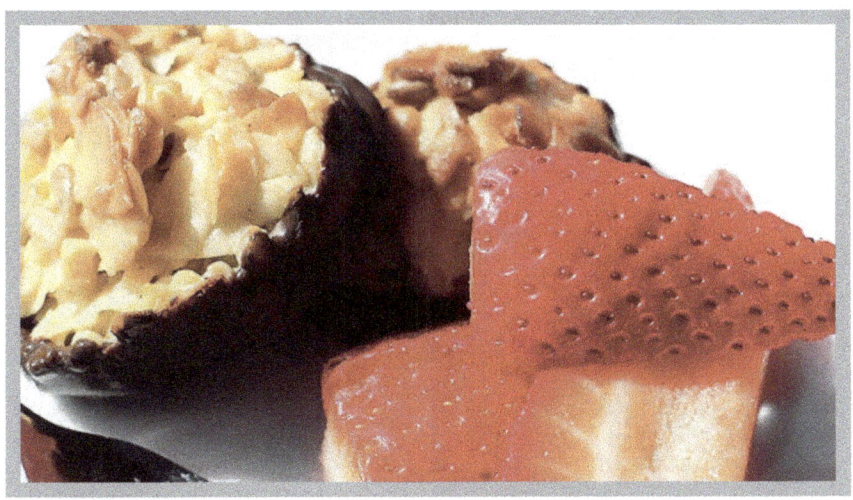

PREPARATION
INGREDIENTS

Put the xylitol, butter and cream in a saucepan and bring to a boil. Let it simmer for about 5 minutes.

Add the flaked almonds, sunflower seeds, chopped almonds,

orange zest and cinnamon and simmer for another 5 minutes. Mix well over and over again.

Remove the mixture from the heat and let it cool slightly.

Prepare a muffin bowl for 12 muffins and distribute the mixture evenly on top. Finally press firmly on every single Florentine.

Pre-heat oven to 180 ° C and bake the low carb Florentines for about 5 minutes until golden brown.

Then let it cool completely in the mold. (Preferably overnight).

Finally, melt the sugar-free chocolate in a saucepan (or in a bain-marie) over low heat and garnish the low-carb Florentines with it.

Preparation time: approx. Minutes

SERVINGS: for 12 pieces (one muffin mold)

SOFT LOW CARB COOKIES WITH CHOCOLATE CHIPS

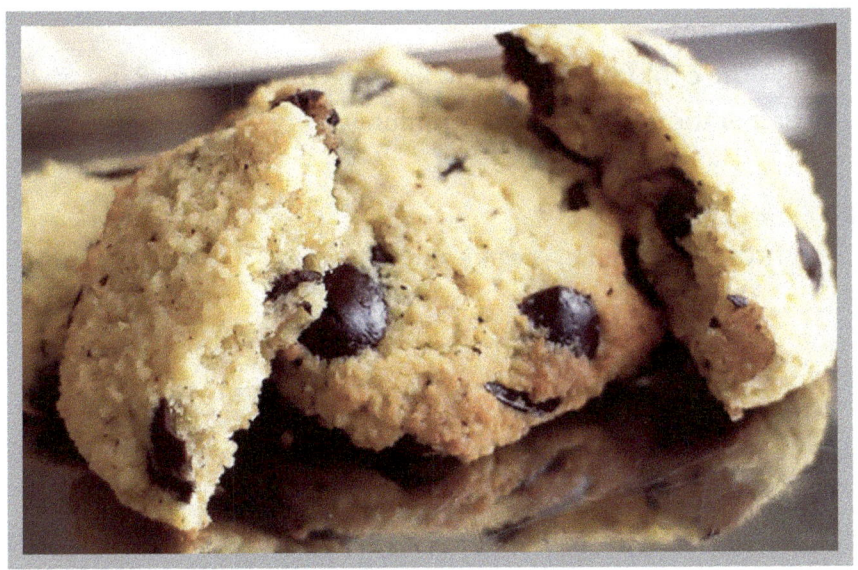

PREPARATION
INGREDIENTS

Preheat the oven to 150 ° C.

Separate the eggs and beat two egg whites in a large bowl until firm.

Put the egg yolks (4 pieces) in a second bowl.

Slowly melt the coconut oil and butter in a small saucepan over low heat.

Let it cool a little and add the egg yolk together with the almond flour, coconut flour and vanilla and mix until you get a homogeneous mixture.

Finally introduce the chocolate chips and stir in the well beaten egg white.

Form a biscuit with half a spoonful of dough in your hand, lift it from the palm of your hand with a knife and place it on a baking sheet lined with parchment paper.

Bake the low-carb cookies in the preheated oven for about 15-20 minutes.

Let the cookies cool for the flavor to develop properly.

Preparation time: about 35 minutes.

SERVINGS: for about 20 cookies.

4
LOW CARB PEANUT COOKIES WITH WHOLE PEANUTS

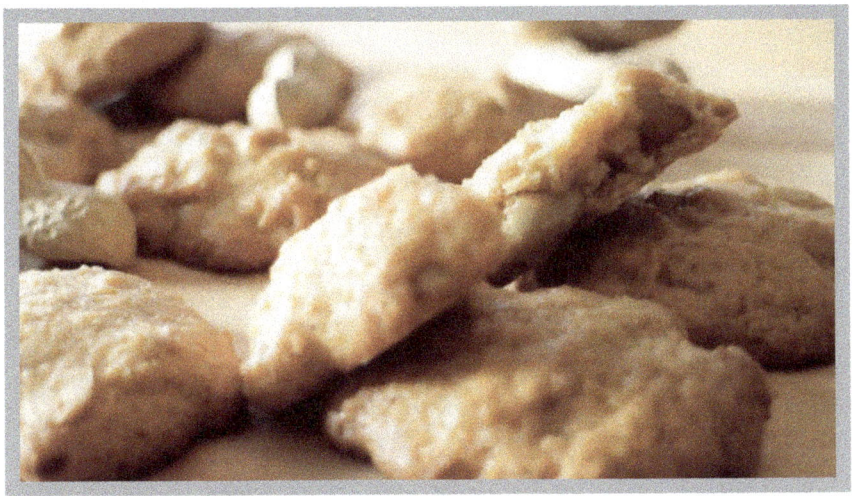

PREPARATION
INGREDIENTS

Preheat the oven above / below to 170 ° C.
Mix the peanut butter, xylitol, and an egg well in a bowl.

Now add the whole peanuts and coconut flour and season with salt.

Use two half tablespoons of the batter to spread small spots on a parchment paper lined baking sheet.

Bake the low carb peanut cookies for about 10-15 minutes at 170 °C on top / bottom.

Let cool well.

Preparation time: approx. 20 minutes.

SERVINGS: **Makes 10 peanut crackers**

LOW CARB CHRISTMAS PUMPKIN SPICE SLICES WITH ORANGE FROSTING

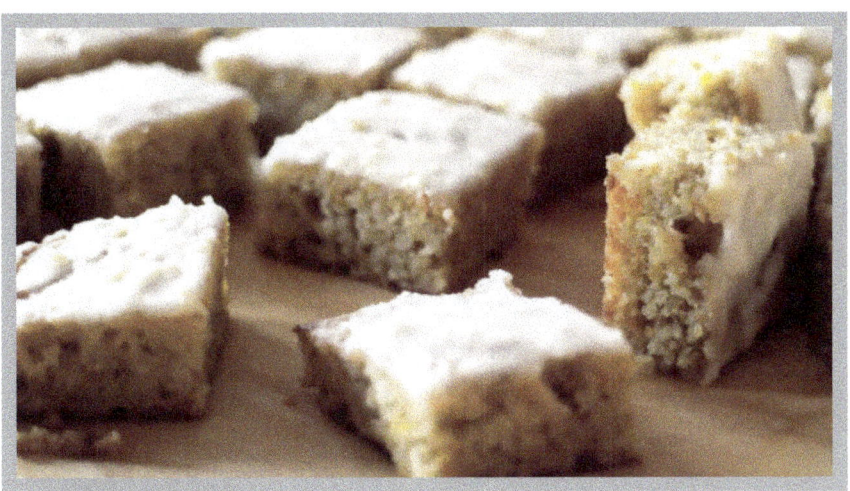

PREPARATION
INGREDIENTS

Wash the pumpkin, grate it coarsely with a kitchen grater and place in a bowl.

Beat the eggs, add 100 g of xylitol and mix everything well.

and heat butter in a saucepan over low heat and let it cool slightly.

Now add the almond flour, psyllium husk, baking powder, and butter.

Finely chop the cardamom, cinnamon and cloves with a mortar and pestle and mix well.

Place the dough on a parchment lined baking sheet and roll it out to a height of about 1cm.

Bake the low carb pumpkin spice slices at 160 ° C over / under heat for about 30 minutes and let cool.

Mix 70 g in a small bowl, crush into powder, xylitol, orange peel and lemon juice and distribute over the cooked noodles.

Once the orange glaze has solidified, use a knife to cut the batter into cubes.

Low Carb Pumpkin Slices with Orange Frosting pair wonderfully with the holiday season.

Preparation time: approx. 50 minutes.

Servings: for about 60 spice cubes.

6

LOW CARB JAM COOKIES (HUSSAR DONUTS)

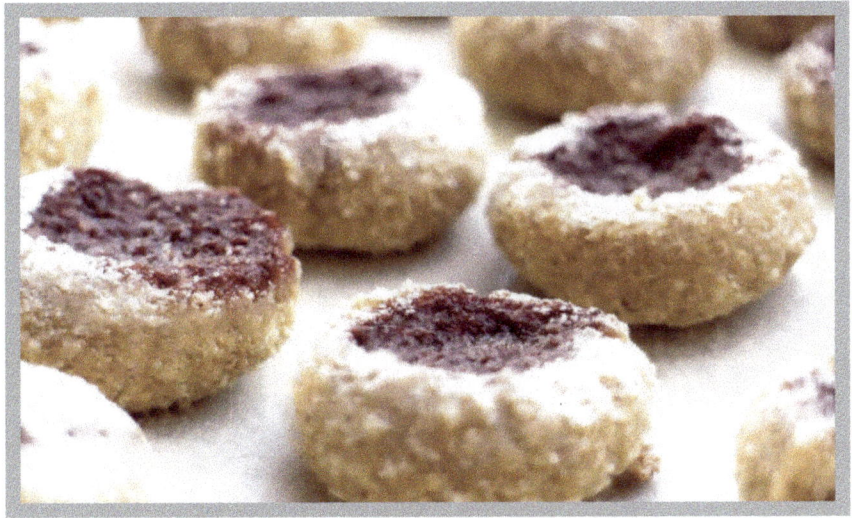

PREPARATION
INGREDIENTS

In a bowl, mix the xylitol and eggs well.
In a second bowl, mix the almond flour, coconut flour, psyl-

lium husk, baking powder, vanilla and a pinch of salt and add to the egg and xylitol mixture.

Stir with a spoon and let it rest for about 5 minutes.

Now add the butter to the dough and knead until smooth with your hands.

Roll a teaspoon of dough into a ball in each hand and make a hole with your thumb.

Fill the cookies with the jam without added sugar and bake them in the oven at 160 °C high / low for about 15 minutes.

Let the low carb jam cookies cool well and sprinkle with powdered xucker if desired.

Preparation time: approx. 35 minutes.

SERVINGS: approx. 36 pieces.

7
LINZER BISCUITS WITH JAM (LOW CARB)

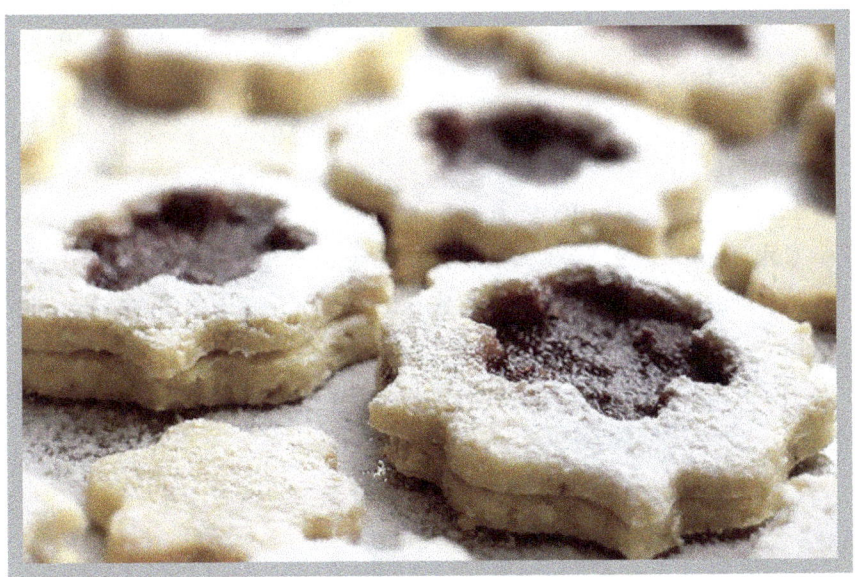

PREPARATION
INGREDIENTS
heat the butter in a saucepan over low heat and set aside.

Combine the xylitol, eggs, and slightly cold butter in a large bowl.

In a second bowl, mix together the almond flour, coconut flour, baking powder, carob seed flour, vanilla and a pinch of salt.

Now add the flour mixture to the egg-xylitol-butter mixture and knead until smooth.

Form the dough into a ball, wrap it in cling film and refrigerate for 15-30 minutes.

Sprinkle the counter with almond flour and roll out the dough into small portions. The dough should be sprinkled with a little almond flour on both sides. and This will make it easier to roll out and the dough will not stick to the roll.

Cut the rolled dough with a large cookie cutter (see photo). Repeat the same operation with the pasta left over from the cut.

Now count the cookies and cut half of the cookies into a smaller shape (see B).

Brush the perforated biscuits with unsweetened jam and lay the cut biscuits on top twice.

Finally, fill the hole with the jam.

Bake the Linz Low Carb Biscuits at 150 ° C upper / lower temperature in the oven for about 15-20 minutes and then let them cool very well.

Sprinkle with xylitol powder or xylitol powder as desired and enjoy.

Preparation time: about 55 minutes

SERVINGS: about 25 cookies.

LOW-CARB SHORTBREAD COOKIES WITH LEMON GLAZE

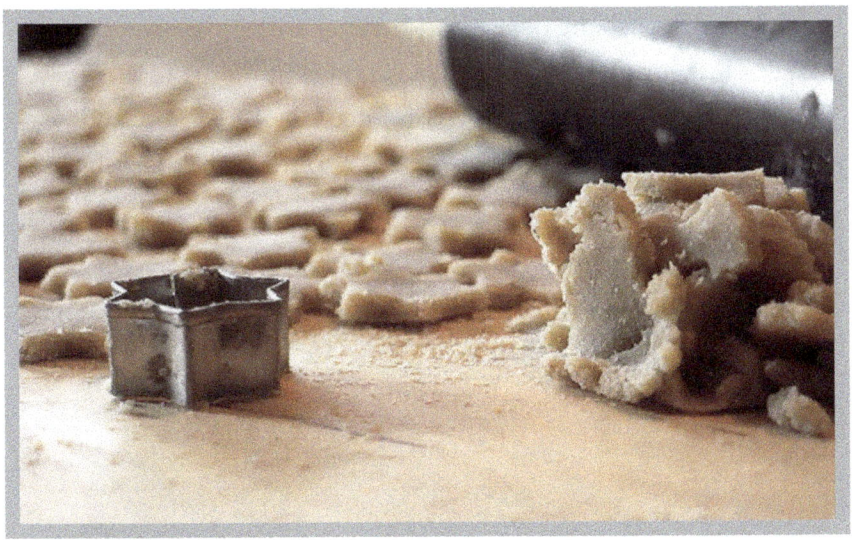

PREPARATION
INGREDIENTS
break the eggs, pour them in a bowl and beat.
Add xylitol and mix.

Then add the almond flour, coconut flour, baking powder, carob seed flour, vanilla and a pinch of salt and mix well with a spoon.

Weigh and add the butter at room temperature and mix everything with your hands until it forms a homogeneous mixture.

make Shape the dough into a ball, wrap it in cling film and let it rest in the refrigerator for about 30 minutes.

Cut a piece of dough and flatten it in your hands. Sprinkle the work surface and the dough (on both sides) with almond flour.

Now carefully roll out the dough and cut it. As soon as the dough sticks, sprinkle some almond flour again.

Place the low carb shortbread cookies on a baking sheet lined with parchment paper and bake them in the oven at 160 ° C high / low for about 15 minutes. Then let them cool well.

Mix the lemon juice with the juice of one lemon and some xucker powder and spread it over the cookies with a brush.

Preparation time: about 100 minutes.

SERVINGS: for a pan.

9
LOW CARB LEMON HEARTS (CHRISTMAS COOKIES)

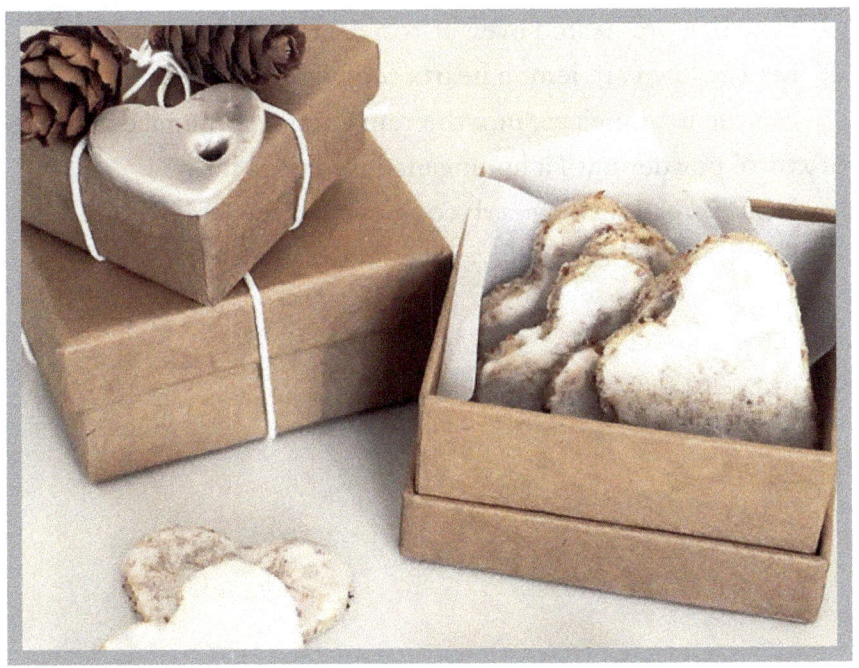

PREPARATION

INGREDIENTS

In a big bowl, and whisk the egg whites till firm.

Use a coffee grinder or mortar to grind the xylitol into powder. Alternatively, you can use Xucker powder.

Rub 60g of xylitol powder into hard egg white and continue beating.

Add two teaspoons of lemon juice, one teaspoon of lemon zest and chopped almonds and mix well.

and Shape into a ball and leave to rest in the refrigerator for 30 minutes, covered.

shape the dough to a thickness of about 1/2 cm (eg between two sheets of parchment paper).

Cut with a heart-shaped pan and lay them out on a baking sheet lined with parchment paper.

Bake in a pre-heated oven at 100 degrees for 15 minutes.

Let the low-carb lemon hearts cool well.

For the lemon glaze, mix the remaining lemon juice and 30 g of xylitol powder until a homogeneous mass is formed.

Next, spread the low-carb cookies with the lemon glaze.

Preparation time: about 70 minutes.

SERVINGS: about 55 lemon hearts.

10
LOW CARB WHITE CHOCOLATE CHIP CHOCOLATE CHIP COOKIES

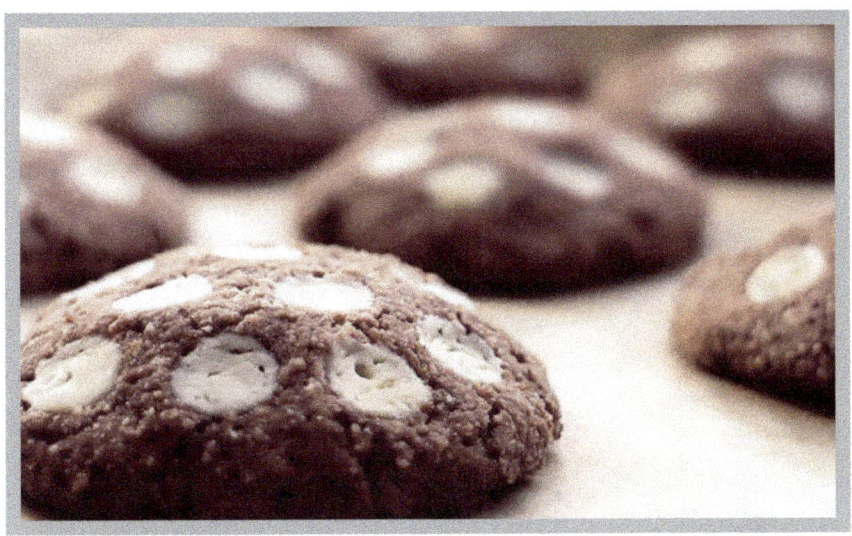

PREPARATION
INGREDIENTS
Mix almond flour, coconut flour, xylitol, cocoa powder,

baking powder, locust bean gum, vanilla and a pinch of salt in a bowl.

In an additional bowl, beat the eggs and add them together with the softened butter.

Work the dough with your hands until it becomes a smooth dough.

Form a cookie with a tablespoon of dough in each hand and place on a parchment paper lined baking sheet.

Finally, press the white chocolate chips into the cookies with the pointy side first.

Bake the Low Carb White Chocolate Chip Chocolate Chip Cookies for about 15 minutes at 155 ° C top / bottom in the oven and cool well.

Preparation time: approx. 40 minutes

SERVINGS: for about 10 cookies.

11
LOW CARB BLACK AND WHITE COOKIES (CHECKERBOARD COOKIES)

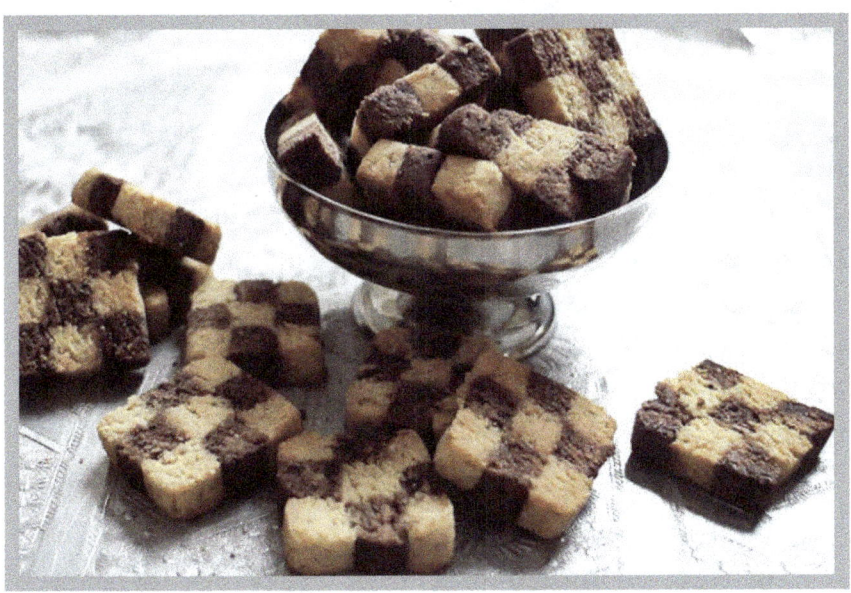

PREPARATION
INGREDIENTS

Combine the almond flour, psyllium husk, xylitol, and vanilla (if desired) in a bowl.

Add the peanut butter, softened butter, and an egg and knead with your hands until a smooth dough forms.

Cut the dough in half and knead a tablespoon of cocoa powder in half.

Shape the light and dark dough into a block with a 3 × 3 cm base and about 15 cm long.

Wrap the two blocks of dough in plastic wrap and place in the freezer for about 15 minutes.

Now cut the dough blocks lengthwise into three pieces. (There are 3 light and 3 dark blocks with the dimensions 1x3x15cm long)

Now we are starting to apply layers for the first time. We start with a piece of light pasta, we put a dark piece on top and then again a piece of light pasta.

We form the second block in reverse order. Dark - light - dark.

Now we have two blocks of dough again, which we process as before, so that in the end a checkerboard pattern is created.

If you're not completely sure how to layer your dough blocks, you can search for the word "checkerboard cookies" on YouTube and read the instructions there.

Finally, cut the checkerboard-shaped dough blocks into slices about 0.5 - 1 cm thick and place them on a parchment paper lined baking sheet.

Bake the low carb black and white cookies for about 15 minutes at 150 ° C top / bottom.

Let cool and store in a cookie jar.

Preparation time: approx. 50 minutes.

. . .

SERVINGS: for approximately 33 cookies.

12
LOW CARB CHOCOLATE ALMOND CLOUDS

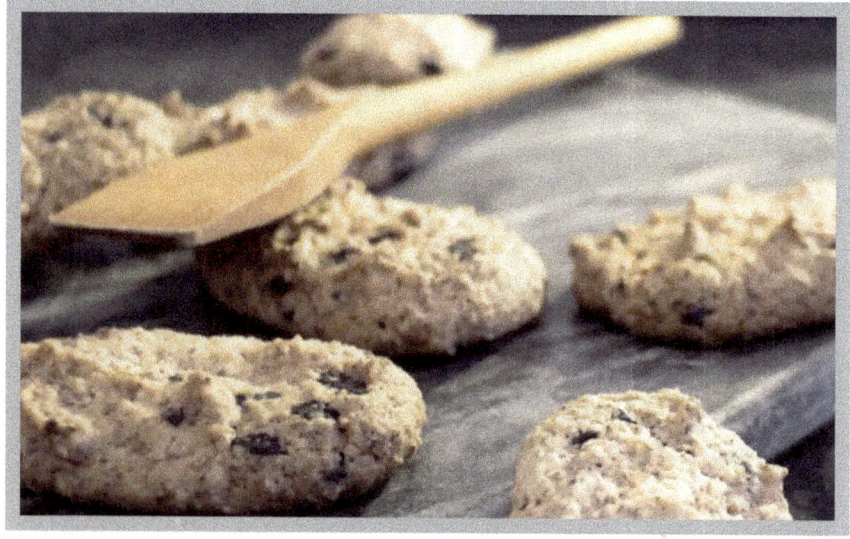

PREPARATION
INGREDIENTS

Beat the egg white very well, slowly pour in the xylitol and the orange peel and continue beating.

Finely chop the chocolate chips and add to the mixture along with the chopped almonds.

Line a baking sheet with parchment paper and use a teaspoon of batter to form elongated clouds on the parchment paper.

Bake in a preheated 150 ° C oven for about 15-20 minutes.

Let cool well and store cookies in cookie jar.

Preparation time: approx. 30 minutes.

SERVINGS: approx. 15 pieces

13

LOW CARB CARROT AND CINNAMON COOKIES

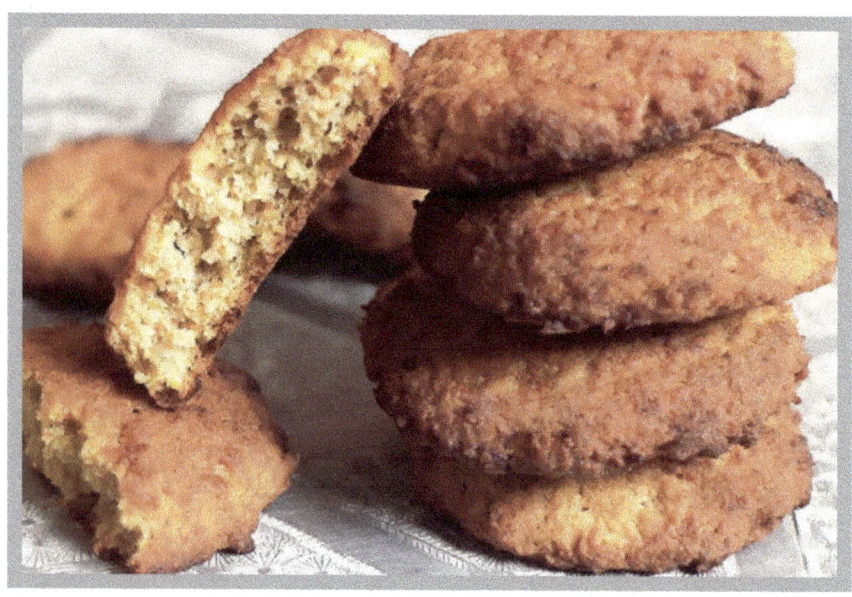

PREPARATION
INGREDIENTS

In a small saucepan, melt the butter over low heat.

In a food processor, whisk together the eggs, xylitol, and butter until frothy.

Peel and grate the carrots with a potato grater.

COMBINE THE ALMOND FLOUR, psyllium husks, baking powder, cinnamon, and nutmeg zest in a separate dish.

To make a homogeneous dough, combine the grated carrot and flour mixture with the xucker egg mixture. Allow the dough to rest for 5 minutes.

Use your hands to shape a cookie out of a tablespoon of dough and put it on a baking sheet lined with parchment paper. (Please note that the dough is very sticky.) The cookies become very fluffy as a result of this, but they are also more difficult to process.)

Preheat the oven to 160 degrees Celsius and bake the low carb cinnamon carrot cookies for about 30 minutes.

Then allow to cool absolutely. The cookies taste better the longer they are steeped.

Time to prepare: about 45 minutes

Approximate serving size: 12 cookies

14
EASY LOW CARB PEANUT COOKIES

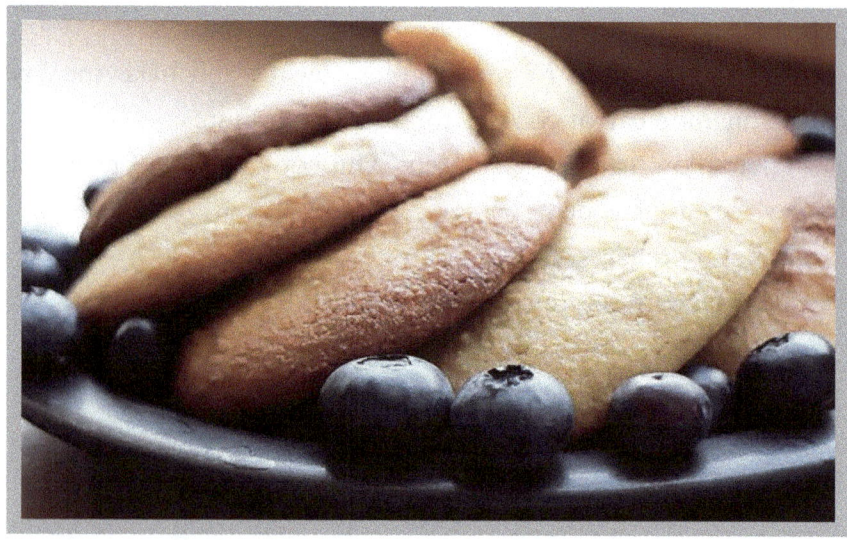

PREPARATION
INGREDIENTS
　Consider: As always, we've crafted the recipe to ensure that

the cookies aren't too sweet. If you want your peanut biscuits to be a little sweeter, add a little more xylitol or erythritol.

Preheat the oven to 150 degrees Celsius in a fan oven.

In a mixing bowl, combine the peanut butter, xylitol, milk, and an egg.

Now apply the psyllium husks and sieve in the coconut flour, mixing it together evenly.

Add a little water at a time before the dough becomes viscous. Line a baking sheet with parchment paper and put a tablespoon of dough on the parchment paper, leaving enough space for each one. The amount of dough we used yielded seven cookies.

Bake the low-carb peanut cookies at 150°C for about 15 minutes, or until golden brown.

To eat, top with blueberries.

Time to prepare: approximately 25 minutes

Approximately 7 cookie servings

15
LOW CARB HAZELNUT CHOCOLATE COOKIES

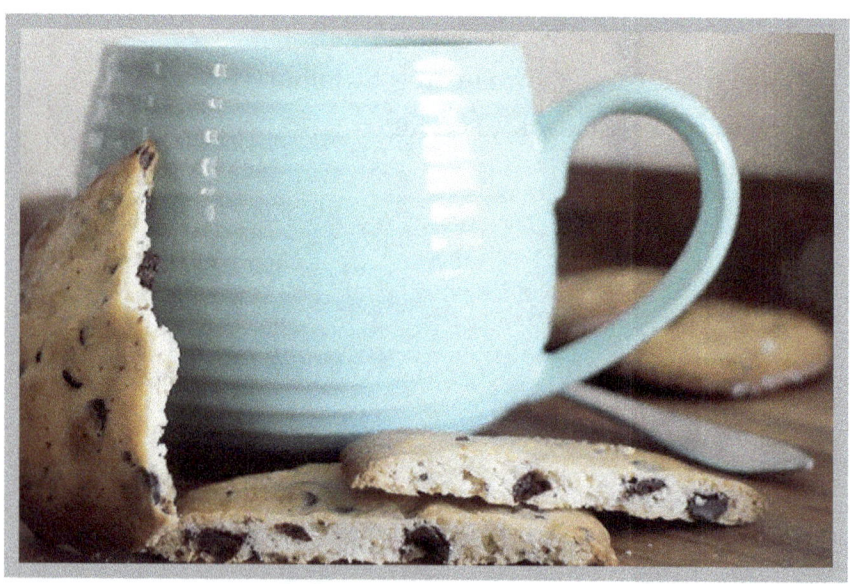

PREPARATION
INGREDIENTS

Heat the oven to 170 degrees Celsius with convection.

In a large mixing bowl, combine the almond butter (also known as cashew butter), xylitol, and an egg to create a smooth mass.

Combine the ground hazelnuts and chocolate chips in a mixing bowl. Allow the dough to rest for a few minutes.

Using two teaspoons, shape approx. 12 cookies on a baking sheet lined with parchment paper. (Tip: Since the dough is very runny, keep the biscuits on the baking sheet separated.)

Bake at 170°C convection for around 10 minutes. Then set it aside to cool and enjoy.

Time to prepare: approximately 20 minutes

12 BISCUITS (approximately) (cookies)

16
LOW CARB CASHEW COCONUT COOKIES (QUICK TO MAKE)

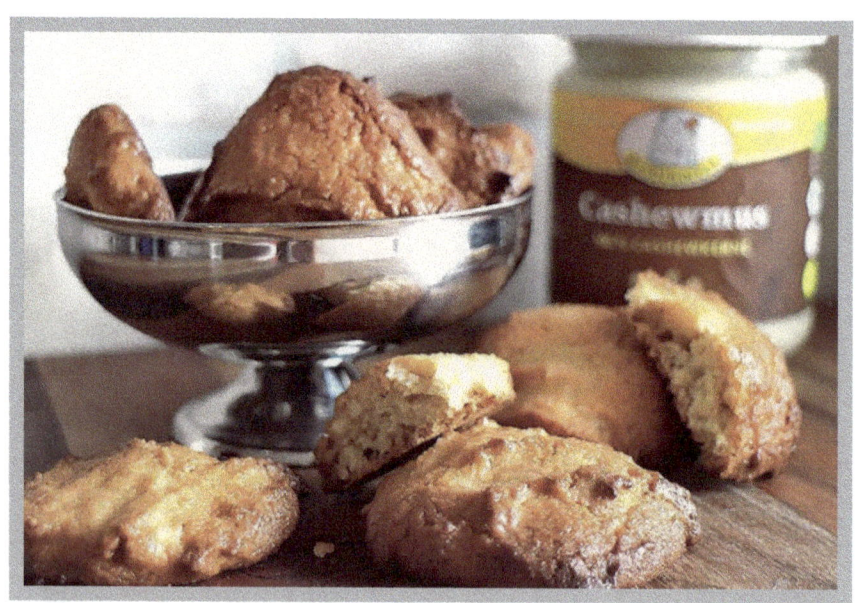

PREPARATION
   INGREDIENTS
   NUTRITIONAL VALUES

Preheat the oven to 170 degrees Celsius in a fan oven.

In a mixing bowl, combine the cashew butter, xylitol, and an egg. Whisk with a fork until the mixture is homogeneous.

Then, using up to 20g coconut flour, bind the cashew mass.

Form half a tablespoon of dough into cookies on a baking sheet lined with baking paper with two tablespoons.

Preheat the oven to 170°C and bake the cookies for about 10-15 minutes, or until golden brown.

Low-carb cookies are simple to make with just a few ingredients and still taste delicious.

Time to prepare: approximately 20 minutes

14 cookies (approximately)

17
LOW CARB CHOCOLATE COCONUT CUBES

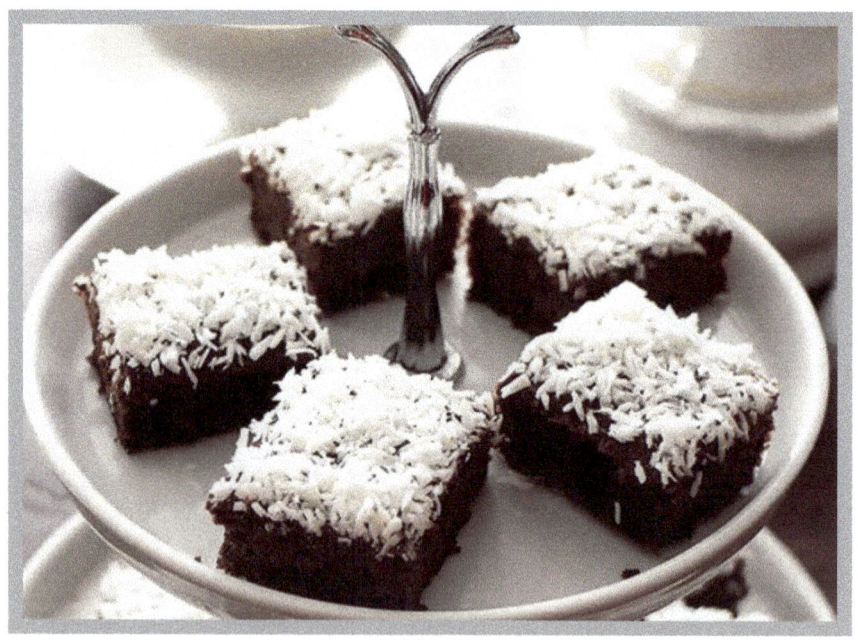

PREPARATION
INGREDIENTS

Split the eggs and beat the egg whites until stiff in a mixing bowl. Melt the butter and coconut oil in a low-temperature water bath.

In a separate cup, whisk together the egg yolks, melted butter and coconut oil, boubon vanilla, cocoa powder, and xylitol until light and fluffy.

To make a smooth dough, blend the almond flour and baking powder, fold into the mixture, and add 4 tablespoons of hot water. Fold in the egg whites gradually and carefully.

Line a baking sheet with baking paper, spread the dough over an area of approximately 20cm x 26cm, and bake for 35 minutes at 160° C top / bottom heat.

Allow for complete cooling of the base.

Melt the chocolate in a water bath by breaking it into bits. Apply the liquid chocolate to the baked foundation with a brush. Chocolate can be used to cover the entire surface.

Sprinkle the desiccated coconut uniformly over the base and set aside until the chocolate has hardened again.

Last but not least, break the base into cubes or rectangles and enjoy.

Time to prepare: approximately 90 minutes

Approximate serving size: 20 bits

LOW CARB CINNAMON STARS (APPROX. 30 PIECES)

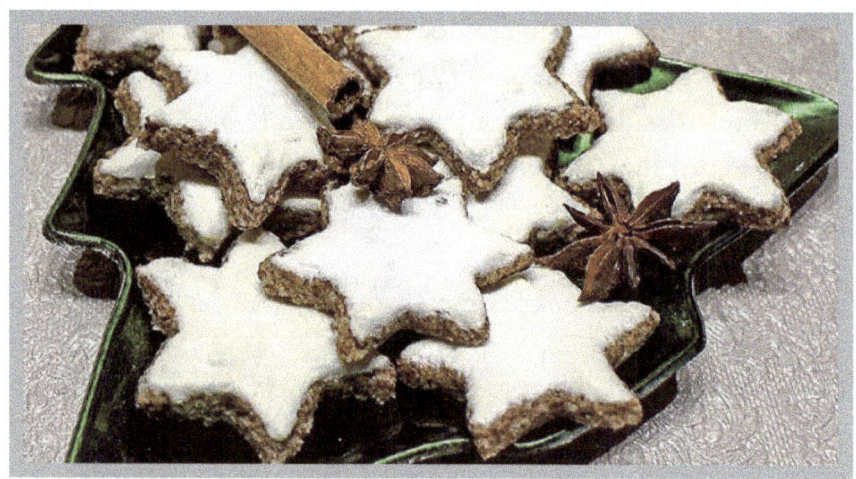

PREPARATION
INGREDIENTS

Egg whites should be rigid. Continue to beat in the lemon juice and birch sugar until the birch sugar has dissolved in the egg white.

3 tablespoons egg whites, set aside

Stir in the remaining egg whites with a spoon (not a mixer!) after mixing the hazelnuts, almonds, and cinnamon.

Allow for a 20-minute cooling period in the refrigerator.

Remove the dough and roll it out to the perfect thickness between two baking papers before cutting out the stars. (Tip: keep the mold submerged in warm water.)

Brush with the remaining egg whites and bake for 12 minutes on the lowest rack in a preheated oven at 140 degrees.

Time to prepare: about 60 minutes

Servings: The dough yields approximately 30

19
LOW CARB COCONUT MACAROONS

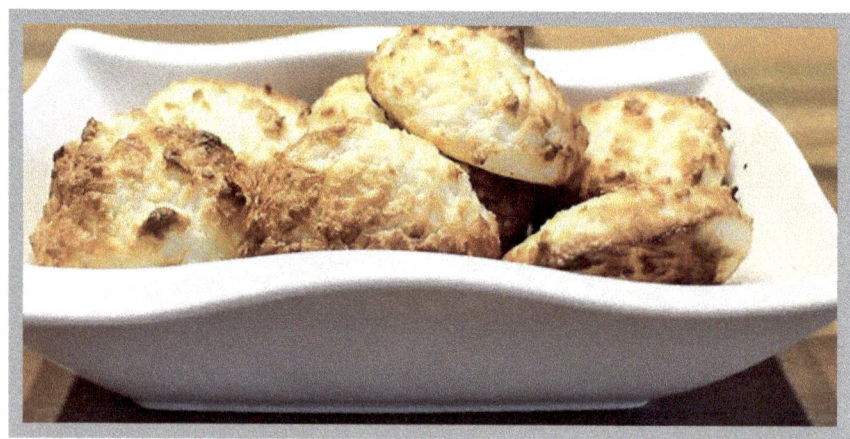

PREPARATION
INGREDIENTS

Using an electric mixer, stiffen the egg whites. Allow the xylitol to slowly drip in and continue to beat until the xylitol has fully dissolved.

Mix well with the quark and coconut flakes.

Pile the macaroons on a baking sheet lined with baking paper using two spoons.

Bake for about 10 minutes at 175 degrees.

The finished coconut macaroons will be around 14 in number.

Time to prepare: approximately 20 minutes

Approximate number of servings: 14

20
LOW CARB GINGERBREAD COOKIES WITH CHOCOLATE ICING

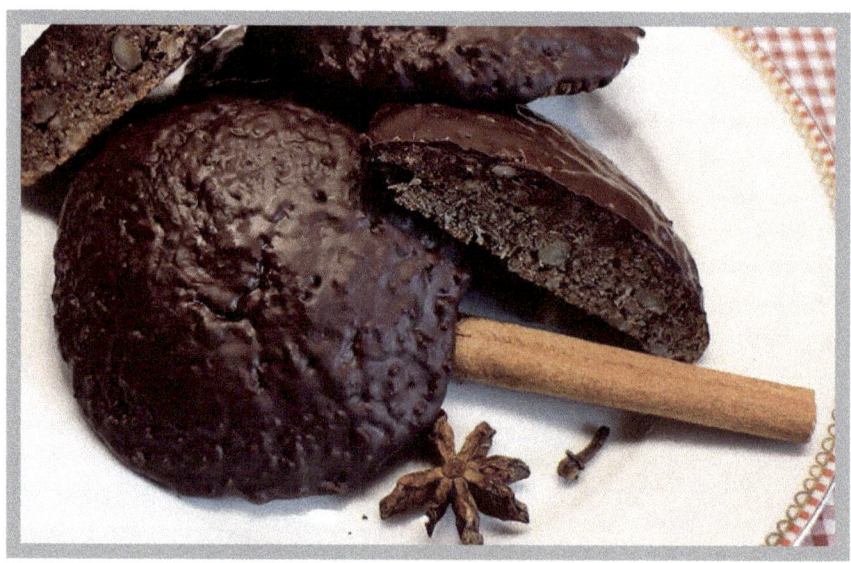

PREPARATION
   INGREDIENTS
   Combine the almond flour, ground hazelnuts, chopped hazel-

nuts, chopped almonds, birch sugar, honey, and spices in a big mixing bowl.

3 eggs, beaten until foamy in a food processor, and stirred into the mixture

Preheat the oven to 170 degrees Fahrenheit on the top and bottom racks, and let the dough rest for 5 minutes.

Make 5 gingerbread cookies with the dough and put them on a baking sheet lined with parchment paper.

Preheat the oven to 350°F and bake the gingerbread for 20 minutes.

Remove the gingerbread from the oven and set aside to cool for a few minutes.

Warm the chocolate in a water bath and use a brush to glaze the gingerbread. (Add a splash of cream and a pinch of birch sugar if the chocolate is too bitter for you.)

Time to prepare: roughly 40 minutes

5 big gingerbread cookies (servings)

21

LOW CARB APPLE AND CINNAMON COOKIES

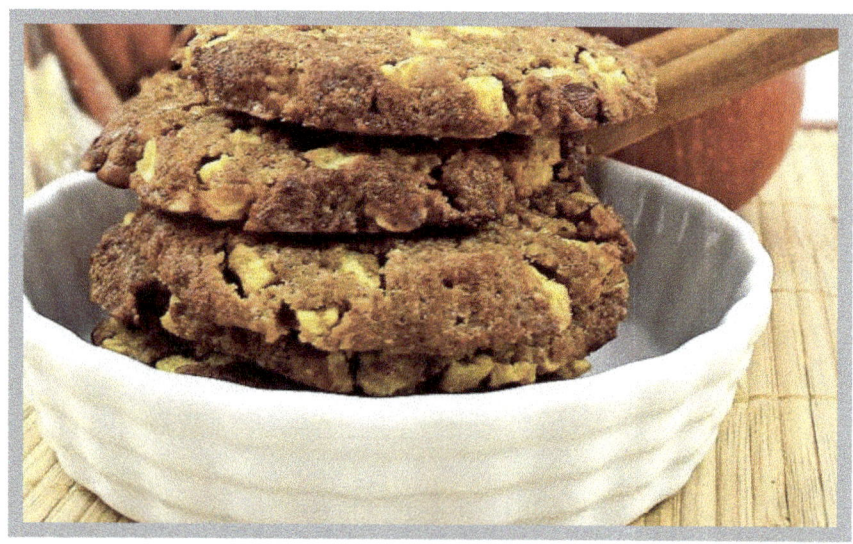

PREPARATION
INGREDIENTS

In a small saucepan over low heat, slowly melt the butter.

Allow the butter to cool slightly before mixing it with the egg yolks.

Remove the core from the apple and dice it finely. Cut the walnuts into small parts with a knife.

Combine almond flour, xylitol (an alternative to Erytritol), cinnamon, apple bits, and walnuts in a mixing bowl.

Preheat oven to 150 degrees Fahrenheit (convection).

Preheat the oven to 350°F and line a baking sheet with parchment paper.

Roll out a teaspoon of dough into a ball in your hands and form into a cookie.

12-15 minutes should be enough time to bake the low carb apple and cinnamon cookies.

Then set it aside to cool and enjoy.

Time to prepare: approximately 35 minutes

22
WINTER LOW CARB COCONUT MACAROONS

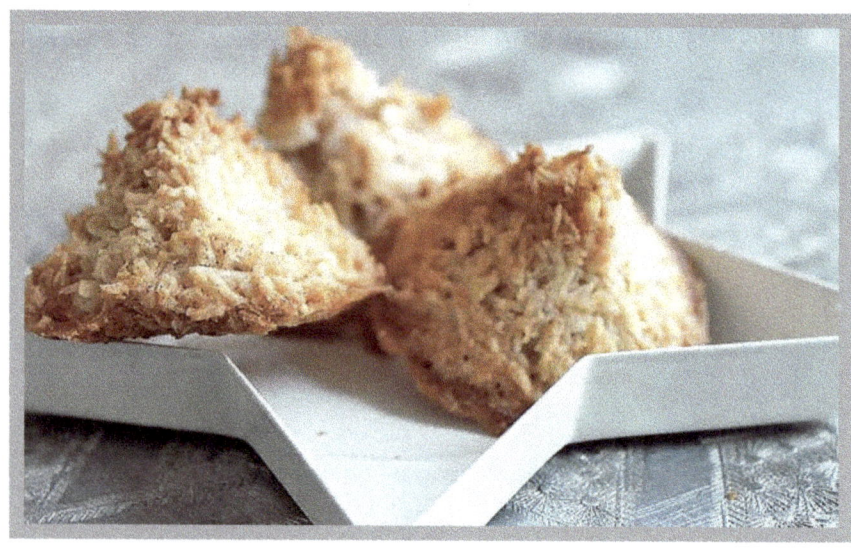

PREPARATION
INGREDIENTS
Heat the oven to 130 degrees Celsius. 4 egg whites, whisked

until stiff Fold in the remaining ingredients one at a time under the egg whites, keeping the dough malleable.

On a greased plate, make tiny mountains with two spoons. Preheat the oven to 200°F and bake for 20-25 minutes.

Allow the macaroons to cool completely before storing them in an airtight container in a biscuit box.

Time to prepare: 10 minutes plus 25 minutes of baking

Time to prepare: approximately 35 minutes.

㉓ COOKIES TO RASPBERRY CHEESECAKE

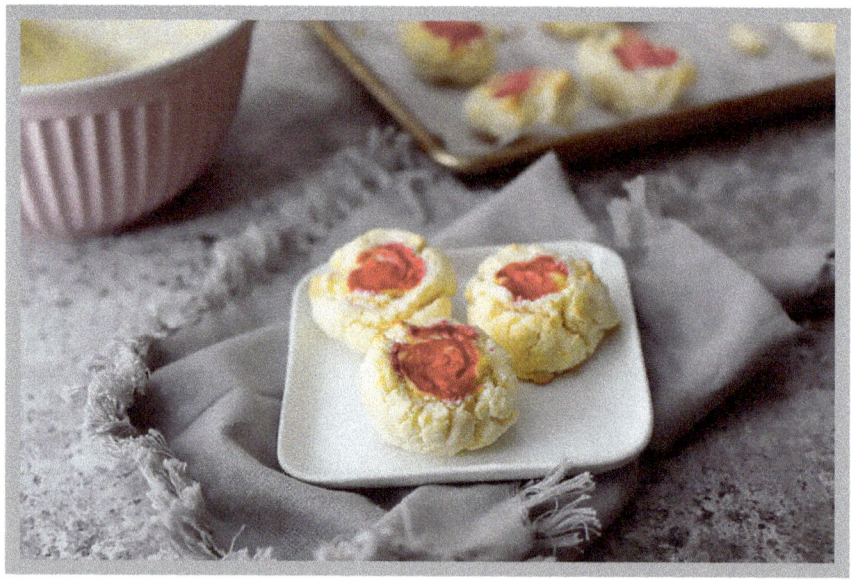

READINESS
  Filling with framboises
  3 Ounces of framboises

1 1/2 cubic lbs of erythritol powder

Filling with cream cheese

4 Ounces of crème fraîche

2 Powdered spoonfuls of erythritol

Extract 1/2 Teaspoon Vanilla

1/2 big ovum

Cookie Teak

One and a half cup of melted butter

1 Ounce of soft cheese

1/2 cup of powdered erythritol

1/2 big ovum

1 Vanilla Teaspoon Extract

2 1/2 cups of almond blanched flour

Preparing

Preheat oven until 350F. Line a parchment-papered baking sheet. Place in a blender and puree the raspberries and erythritol powder until smooth. To filter the seeds of the raspberry using a mesh sieve.

And let raspberry sauce cool down at low heat, and reduce by 1/3. Disable the flame, and let it cool down to room temperature.

For cream cheese filling, using a hand mixer to mix cream cheese, erythritol, egg and vanilla from the ingredients.

In another tub, pound the butter, cream cheese, and cookie-dough ingredients erythritol together.

Combine the vanilla extract and the remaining egg and almond flour together. The dough will crack but it will be able to compress.

Forme the cookie dough into 2 portions of a table spoon and roll into balls. Using a spoon 's back to flatten the batter, and make tiny indoor indentations.

Place some filling with cream cheese in each well, then add a small drop of raspberry puree to each biscuit. Gently whirl around with a toothpick.

Cook 10-15 minutes. The edges are light brown, and continue to build the filling. Let the cookies completely cook before trying to remove them from the oven.

24

LOW CARB SHORTBREAD COOKIES WITH ALMOND FLOUR

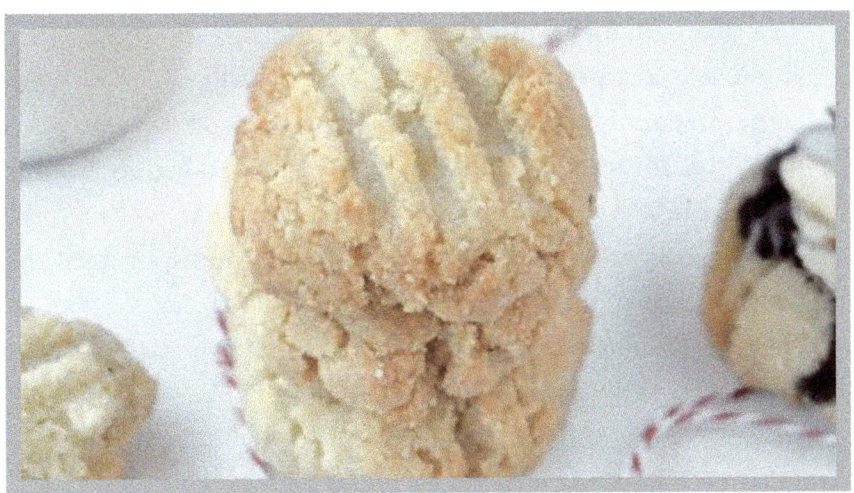

20 MINS

PREPARATION
INGREDIENTS
1 1/3 cup Almond Flour
1/4 cup erythritol

1/4 cup Soft Unsalted Butter at room temperature for 3 hours

1/2 teaspoon Vanilla essence

1/8 teaspoon salt

CHOCOLATE DECORATION - OPTIONAL

1 oz Sugar-free Chocolate Chips

1/2 teaspoon Coconut oil

Preheat the oven to 356 degrees Fahrenheit (180C).

Using parchment paper, line a baking sheet. Delete from the equation.

Mix all of the ingredients together for around 1 minute, or until a cookie crumble forms. An electric mixer or a stand mixer with a hook attachment may be used.

To make a cookie ball, gather the cookie crumble in your hands.

In a tub, chill for 10 minutes.

Remove 1 teaspoon of dough from the fridge and drop it onto the prepared baking sheet, leaving a thumb space between each cookie. You can also make balls out of the dough by rolling it in your hands. After that, gently flatten the cookie with a fork.

Bake the shortbread cookies for 8 to 11 minutes, or until the tops begin to turn golden brown.

Remove from the oven and allow to cool on the baking sheet for 10 minutes before moving to a cooling cookie rack to cool fully before decorating.

DESIGN

In a saucepan, combine the sugar-free chocolate and coconut oil.

Stir and melt the chocolate over medium heat.

Drizzle a little chocolate on some (or all) of the cookies with a scoop.

Cookies can be stored in a cookie jar for up to 3 weeks.

KETO GINGERBREAD COOKIES VEGAN AND GLUTEN-FREE

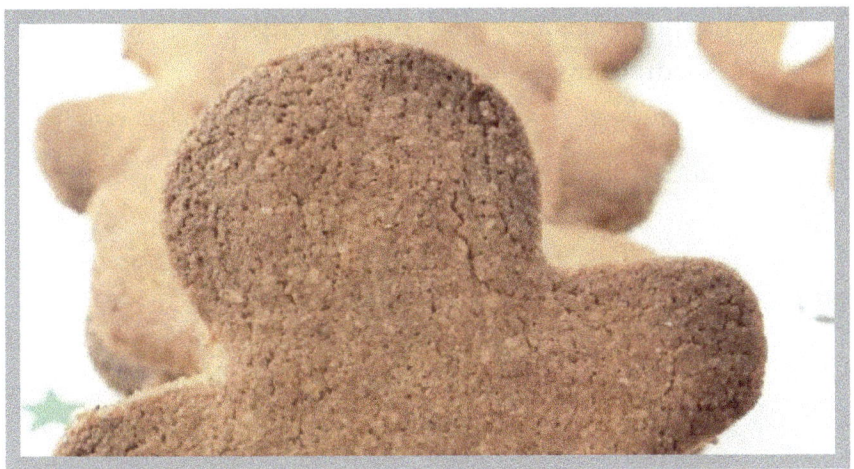

50 mins

PREPARATION
INGREDIENTS
DRY INGREDIENTS

. . .

2 cup Almond Flour or almond meal

1/2 cup Erythritol or golden monk fruit

1 teaspoon Ground ginger

1/2 tablespoon Ground cinnamon

1 teaspoon Baking Powder or 1/2 teaspoon baking soda

1/4 teaspoon ground cloves

WET INGREDIENTS

1 large Egg or 1 tablespoon chia seed + 3 tablespoons water

1/4 cup Coconut oil melted or butter

1 teaspoon Vanilla extract

1 tablespoon black strap molasse - optional, recipe work without it but great iron boost for vegan

KETO ROYAL ICING

1 cup sugar free icing sugar

1-2 tablespoon Unsweetened Almond Milk

1/4 teaspoon guar gum

26
KETO CHOCOLATE SUGAR COOKIES

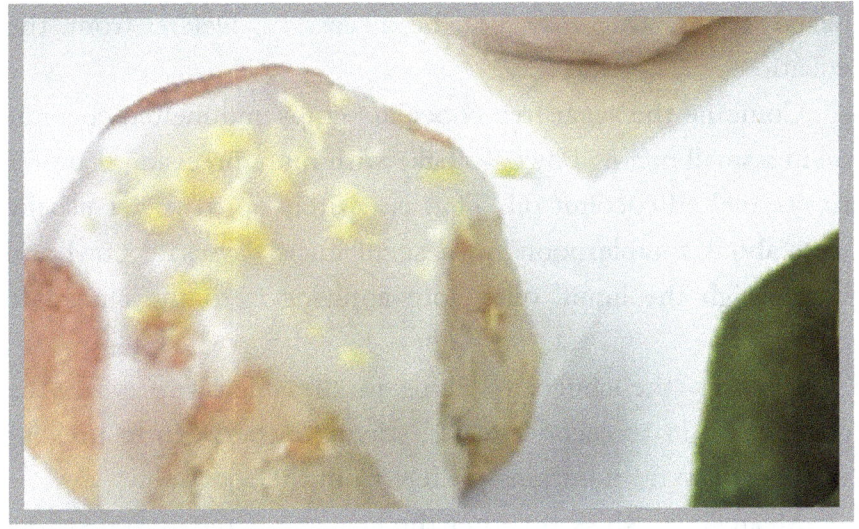

22 mins

PREPARATION
INGREDIENTS

4 ounces Sugar-free Chocolate Chips

2 tablespoon Coconut oil

1 large Egg - at room temperature (or flaxegg if vegan)

1/3 cup Erythritol

1 teaspoon Vanilla essence

1/4 teaspoon Baking Powder

1/4 tespoon salt

1/4 cup Almond Flour

2 teaspoon unsweetened cocoa powder

1/4 cup Pecan nuts - or sugar free chocolate chips

Preheat the oven to 180 degrees Celsius (370F).

Preheat the oven to 350°F and line a baking sheet with parchment paper. If required, spray some oil on the parchment paper; but, depending on how well your parchment paper adheres to baked goods, this may not be necessary. Delete from the equation.

Combine the sugar-free chocolate chips and melted coconut oil in a small mixing bowl. To bake with more precision, I prefer to use melted coconut oil. That is entirely up to you; I usually melt about 2 tablespoons in a small microwave-safe bowl and then weigh the liquid oil before applying it to the chocolate chips.

Heat up the chocolate chips in the microwave with the coconut oil in 30-second bursts, stirring in between to prevent the chocolate from burning. Delete from the equation.

Meanwhile, whisk together the egg, sugar-free crystal sweetener, vanilla essence, baking powder, and salt in a medium mixing bowl. It should take no more than 20 seconds to complete.

Combine the molten chocolate and the remaining ingredients in a mixing bowl. The mixture will thicken and remain shiny, which is just what you want.

POUR in the unsweetened cocoa powder and almond flour. It should only take a minute to completely integrate anything with a spoon. To stop the batter drying out, don't overmix it. The batter will thicken again, resembling brownie batter in nature, dense but still runny. If your almond flour is coarse (also known as almond meal), you can see some small bits of almond flour, which is fine.

Depending on your preference, stir in the sliced pecan nuts or chocolate chips.

POUR THE BATTER onto the cookie sheet that has been prepared. From this dough, you should be able to make 6 big cookies. Since the cookies can expand significantly during baking, leave about 4 cm between each cookie. On my cookie sheet, I made two rows of three cookies.

COOK FOR 10-14 MINUTES, or until the edges are golden brown. It's natural for the middle to remain soft. For a brownie texture, I considered 12 minutes to be ideal. Remove the cookie sheet from the oven and set aside to cool for 10 minutes.

Use a spatula to slip under each cookie to prevent them from breaking and place them on a cooling rack. They're always a little soft.

On the shelf, cool down for another 10 minutes.

. . .

KEEP for up to 5 days in a cookie jar. When new, the texture is smooth and similar to that of a brownie. The next day, the texture changes, becoming chewier in the middle and crispier on the edges.

27
NO-BAKE KETO COOKIES

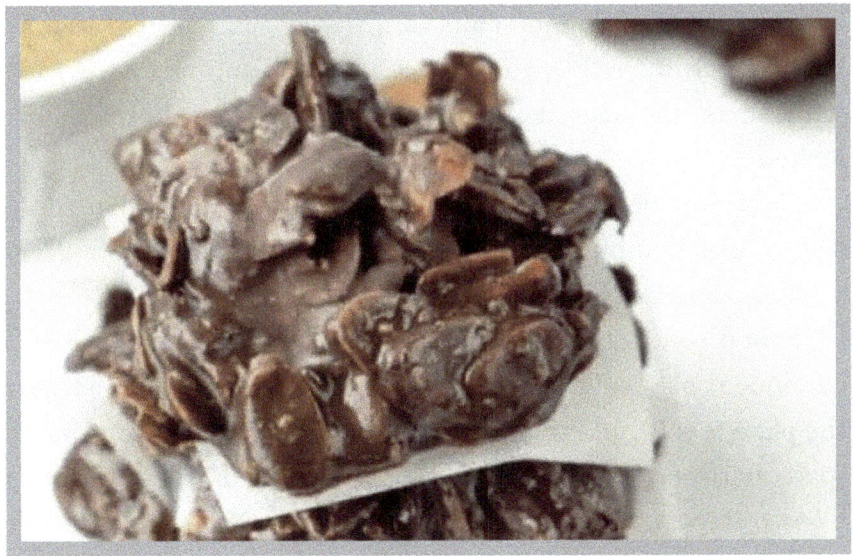

15 mins
PREPARATION
INGREDIENTS

1/3 cup almond butter

1 tablespoon Coconut oil

1/2 cup Sugar-free Chocolate Chips

1 1/4 cup Sliced almonds

1 tablespoon Chia seeds

Using parchment paper, cover a big plate or chopping board. When you're making the cookie batter, put the plate in the fridge.

Combine almond butter, coconut oil, and sugar-free chocolate chips in a microwave-safe dish (or bars chopped in small pieces).

To stop burning the almond butter, microwave in 30-second bursts, stirring in between. All of your ingredients should be thoroughly combined in no more than 90 seconds.

Place all of the ingredients in a small saucepan if you don't have a microwave. Place over medium heat and mix constantly until all of the ingredients are mixed and the chocolate has melted.

Combine the sliced almonds and chia seeds in a mixing dish. The chocolate mixture should fully cover the almonds and seeds.

Take the plate out of the freezer and set it aside.

Spoon some cookie batter onto the chilled plate lined with parchment paper. The cookie should not expand too far because the plate is cold, and the base should set quickly. Enable 1 thumb space between each cookie in case it expands slightly during baking. Repeat until there is no more batter. You should be able to make 10 bite-size cookies with this recipe.

Return the plate to the freezer for another 10 minutes, or until the chocolate has hardened and set.

COCONUT FLOUR COOKIES NO SUGAR - LOW-CARB SHORTBREAD

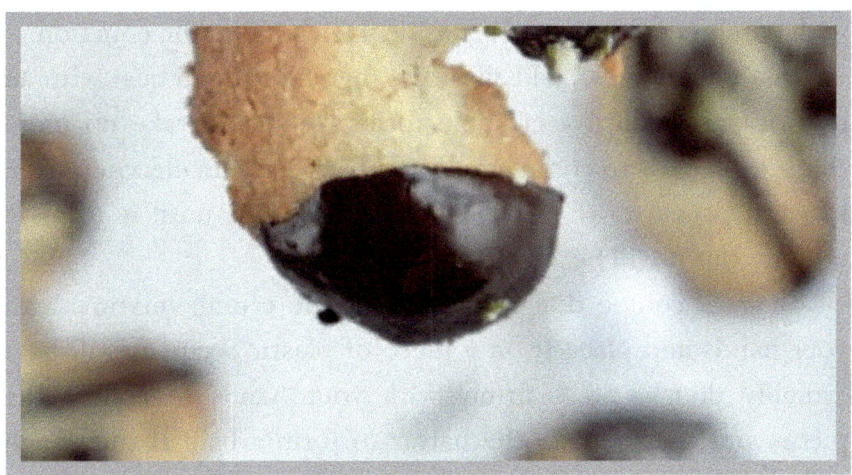

23 mins

PREPARATION
INGREDIENTS

3/4 cup Coconut Flour
1/3 cup Coconut oil solid, not melted +/- 1 tablespoon

1/4 cup Erythritol - monk fruit sugar or erythritol

1/4 teaspoon Vanilla extract

1 large Egg - at room temperature, or 1 tablespoon of peanut butter

DECORATION

1/3 cup Sugar-free Dark Chocolate

1 tablespoon Pumpkin seeds crushed

1 teaspoon unsweetened desiccated coconut

OPTIONAL - TO SPRINKLE ON TOP BEFORE BAKING

1 tablespoon Coconut Flour

HEAT THE OVEN to 180°C (350°F) fan bake. Cover a cookie tray with parchment paper and set aside. Delete from the equation.

In a mixing bowl, add all of the ingredients and beat with an electric mixer until a crumble forms. It should take no more than 20 seconds to complete. If you don't have an electric mixer, you can press/rub the dough with your hands until it forms a crumb - but it will be a little messier!

Shape a cookie dough ball out of the crumb mixture with your hands and place it on a piece of plastic wrap. It will be a crumbly dough; press firmly with your hands to collect the pieces and tightly wrap the batter to form a ball. If the dough still doesn't come together after 1 minute of kneading, add a little more coconut oil, up to 1 tablespoon. To firm up, put in the refrigerator for 15 minutes.

Pull the dough from the fridge and open the plastic wrap; it will be firm but crumbly when you take a piece in your hands, which is fine. As the coconut oil softens, kneading the dough makes it easier to shape balls.

Roll 1 tablespoon of dough into a ball in your hands, pressing firmly. Place the balls on the baking sheet that has been prepared. If you want to make crescent-shaped cookies, follow these directions. To begin, roll the ball into a cylinder and pinch the center to create a crescent shape. The quickest way to make lovely round shortbread cookies is to simply flatten the ball with a fork. Repeat with the remaining dough until 12 cookies have been shaped.

Spray extra coconut flour on top of the cookies before baking if needed.

Bake for 6 to 8 minutes, or until the sides are light golden brown. The cookies will remain soft at this stage, which is normal; do not touch them or attempt to remove them from the tray; they will firm up once completely cold.

Cool for about 30 minutes on the baking sheet before it reaches room temperature. The coconut oil hardens as it cools, resulting in crisp, crumbly shortbread cookies. In the summer, I normally put my baking sheet outside to cool down in. If desired, finish with a drizzle of melted sugar-free chocolate. I used stevia-sweetened dark chocolate.

29
KETO SUGAR COOKIES ONLY 1G NET CARB

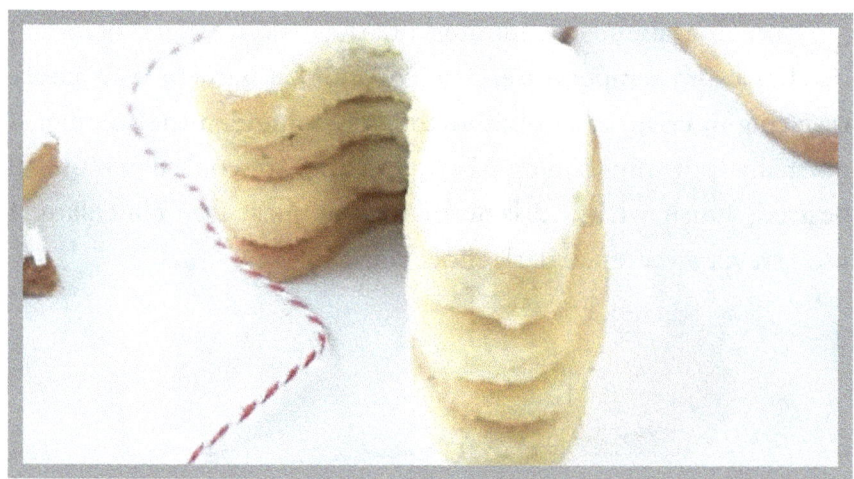

1 HR 27 mins

PREPARATION
INGREDIENTS
1 cup Almond flour
2 tablespoons Coconut flour scooped, packed, level up

1/4 cup Erythritol or use 1/3 cup for very sweet cookies!

1/4 teaspoon Salt

2 oz Unsalted butter soft, cubed into 1/4 inches, at room temperature

1 tablespoon Cream cheese

1 teaspoon Vanilla extract

1/4 teaspoon Almond extract optional

Connect the dry ingredients: almond flour, coconut flour, erythritol, and salt to a food processor fitted with the S blade attachment. Blend on high for 30 seconds to uniformly mix the ingredients. Don't miss this stage because it will pulse the erythritol into a thinner texture.

Stop the food processor and combine the soft butter balls, soft cream cheese, vanilla extract, and almond extract.

REPEAT the process on medium speed until the dough forms big crumbles that can be quickly squeezed and gathered into a dough ball. If your dough is too warm, add an extra tablespoon of almond flour; if it's too dry, add an extra teaspoon of soft cream cheese. Phase for each addition. The dough for the cookies should be fluffy, buttery, and easy to roll into a ball. It should not be too wet or too dry.

Wrap the dough in plastic wrap or place it in a plastic container. Refrigerate for 20 minutes or overnight until flattening into a thick disk.

Preheat the oven to 350°F (180°C) once the dough has cooled. Use parchment paper to line one or two cookie sheets. Delete from the equation.

. . .

PULL the dough disc from the freezer, take off the plastic wrap, and sandwich it between two large sheets of parchment paper. Roll out to a 1/4-inch thickness with a rolling pin. It doesn't matter what shape the rolled dough takes as long as it's 1/4-inch thick. Remove the top piece of parchment paper and use a cookie cutter to cut out cookies from the rolled dough.

Move the cut-out cookies to the prepared cookie sheets using a flat tool, leaving 3 inches between each cookie. In the oven, they will not extend.

Gather the remaining dough into a ball and roll it between the same parchment paper sheets once more.

BAKE COOKIES for 10-12 minutes in the middle rack of your oven, one sheet at a time, until lightly browned around the edges but yellow gold in the center. Since the cookies can cook faster on one side if your oven has hot spots, I suggest rotating the cookie sheet halfway through baking to ensure even baking. When you remove the cookie sheet from the oven, the cookie will be really soft, which is natural!

Cool the cookies on the cookie sheet for 5 minutes before gently sliding a spatula under each cookie and transferring to a cooling rack. After 30 minutes on the rack, they will firm up and achieve their best texture when fully cooled.

30
CHEWY MOLASSES COOKIES

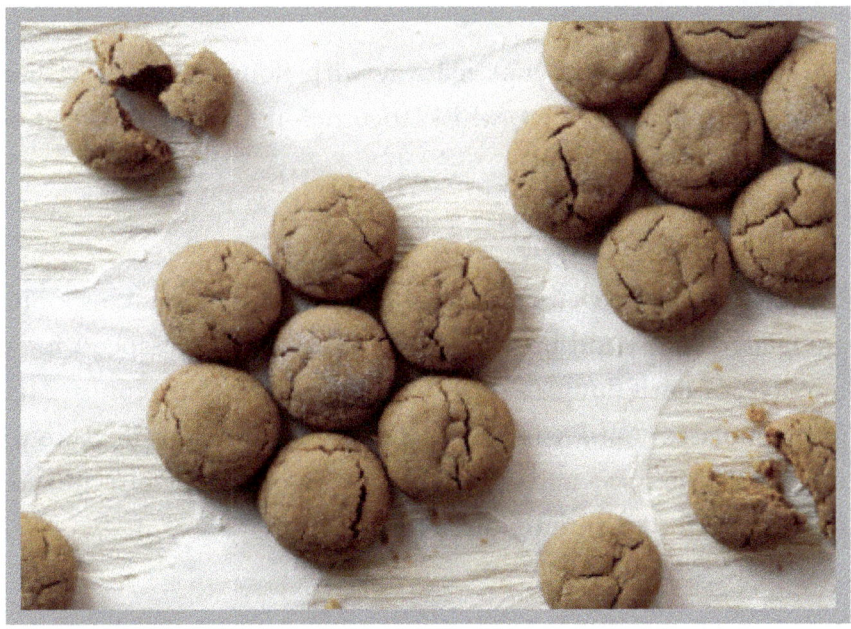

1 HR
PREPARATION

INGREDIENTS

8 ounces all-purpose flour (about 1 3/4 cups)
    1 teaspoon ground cinnamon
    ½ teaspoon baking soda
    ½ teaspoon ground ginger
    ½ teaspoon ground cloves
    ¼ teaspoon baking powder
    ¼ teaspoon salt
    6 tablespoons butter, softened
    8 tablespoons granulated sugar, divided
    ¼ cup dark brown sugar
    1 large egg
    ¼ cup molasses

Fill dry measuring cups halfway with flour and level with a knife. In a mixing bowl, whisk together flour and the next 6 ingredients (through salt).

In a wide mixing bowl, combine the butter, 5 tablespoons granulated sugar, and brown sugar; beat on medium speed for 5 minutes, or until fluffy. Add the egg and beat for 30 seconds. Mix in the molasses until it is fully blended. Add the flour mixture to the butter mixture and blend on low speed until just mixed. Refrigerate for 30 minutes after covering.

Preheat oven to 350 ° degrees Fahrenheit.
    Form dough into 24 balls, each weighing around 1 1/2 tablespoons. Roll remaining 3 tablespoons sugar into balls and put 2

inches apart on parchment-lined baking sheets. Preheat oven to 350°F and bake for 12 minutes, or until set. Cool for 3 minutes on the pan before transferring to a wire rack to cool fully.

Preheat oven to 350°F. BAKE A SECOND BATCH Bake these cookies without a hitch by doubling the dough. To mail, use plastic wrap to wrap small stacks together. Stack in a box with plenty of padding, or in a wide-mouth canning jar with crumpled parchment or wax paper in the headspace underneath the lid. Pack the jar in a box with padding for overnight delivery.

www.ingramcontent.com/pod-product-compliance
Lightning Source LLC
Chambersburg PA
CBHW071124030426
42336CB00013BA/2192